M000087510

POWER
MEGA PUMP
TRANSFORMATION
Method

POWER MEGA PUMP TRANSFORMATION

Method

The Best Isotonic/Isokenetic Exercises that build muscle mass, increase strength, and sculpt the best body Today!

BECOME A POWERFUL MAN!

The Power Mega Pump Transformation Method was written to help you get closer to your physical potential when it comes to real muscle sculpting strengthening exercises. The exercises and routines in this book are quite demanding, so consult your physician and have a physical exam taken prior to the start of this exercise program. Proceed with the suggested exercises and information at your own risk. The Publishers and author shall not be liable or responsible for any loss, injury, or damage allegedly arising from the information or suggestions in this book.

Power Mega Pump Transformation Method
muscle-building Course

By

Birch Tree Publishing
Published by Birch Tree Publishing

Power Mega Pump Transformation Method
Published in 2020, All rights reserved,
No part of this book may be reproduced, scanned,
or distributed in any printed or electronic form without permission.

© 2020 Copyright Birch Tree Publishing
Brought to you by the
Publishers of Birch Tree Publishing
ISBN-978-1-927558-99-7

Birch Tree Publishing

Dedication

To all **VRT** trainees, time to start **GROWING** with self resistance exercises...

Contents

BUILD "POWERFUL" MUSCLES

Introducing the safest physique enhancing series

Introduction by Greg Mangan

Today you can pack on powerful ripped pounds of muscle on your physique in a matter of a few weeks of training. Just think a few pounds of lean muscle mass will make a massive difference on your physique. Even 10 pounds would put the trainee in the superman category. Unfortunately, it takes most trainees some time to gain favorable muscle. However, I am often asked why does the growth process take long most times?
The reason-most trainees do not eat enough which will obstruct the muscle-building process along with workouts that are simply a waste of time.

Those two problems translate into little, and most times zero, muscle growth for extended periods. The Mega Pump Workouts will help you avoid those practices with a solid plan that will push your physique to new levels without wasted effort, as it did for many of my customers. Within these pages contain self resistance strength exercises.

My VRT experience happened in the 80s. It was the result of an experiment with a weightless muscle-stimulating method that I constructed. I have been researching training strategies for building muscle for more than 40 years, which is why I have faith in my VRT system.

The program is a simple one, so please follow it if you want to achieve the best muscle and strength gains possible. However, I must mention that maximum motivation is a must so please give every rep and set your all. Convince yourself that you're going to pack on as much sculpted lean muscle as possible with the training, and as night follows day, you will have just that.

I will continue to research muscle growth, refining the key components of muscle growth that originally spurred the development of a number of effective programs that will follow on within this series. The plan will be to amplify the key muscle-building components—which I have done, as many of my students have packed on more pounds of muscle year after year with the power of VRT training.

So, give the Mega Pump Workouts a shot, and you will be guaranteed a physical transformation—in a matter of weeks. Join the men and women that are already using The VRT programs with great success. **BE TRANSFORMED**.

Yours in Strength and Power

Greg Mangan

LET'S BUILD SOME MUSCLE

LET'S BUILD SOME MUSCLE

If you are reading this book, you already appreciate the importance of exercising for health, strength and wellbeing. The Power Mega Pump Transformation Method will turn you into a powerful well built man. Being a great success at exercising means constant practice to transform yourself to become the best you can be.

When it comes to training-like most everything else in life-sometimes circumstances seem to get in the way from allowing you to exercise. Now, thanks to The Mega Pump Method, you will always get a great workout-no matter where you are.

Resistance strength training with The Power Mega Pump Method enhances:

1) Resistance strength training stimulates muscles to burn more calories than anything else. After your workout your metabolism is triggered for 40 hours after the session.
2) Your body will take on a different shape, and your clothes will fit far better.
3) Your flexibility will increase and resistance training will keep you young.
4) Your bones will become stronger. We lose bone mass as we get older, but resistance strength training increases bone density and add greater strength.
5) A stronger and healthy heart with enhanced blood flow.
6) Stress levels will be reduced due to exercise.
7) Resistance strength training also creates better sleeping patterns.
8) "No need to get depressed". Regular resistance training will ward off symptoms of depression.
9) Mental sharpness will be developed. This takes place due resistance training decreasing blood levels of homocysteine, the protein that's linked to developing Alzheimer's and dementia. Plus, resistance training enhances cognitive function. Workouts will improve memory and you will have longer attention spans.
10) Develop lazar-like focus.

The Strength Training series that will create

a

Muscular

Powerful Body

Chapter 1:
MUSCLE FIBER ANALYSIS

How The Power Mega Pump Isotonic program gives you powerful muscles

Build the body of your dreams with self resistance

01 ABOUT MUSCLE FIBER EFFECTS

There is a lot of rubbish floating around, which leave most more confused about how to build muscle and might. For many years, we were told that 2B fast twitch fibers are best for optimum muscle size.

These are the supposedly get big fibers. Truhfully, the true fibers for muscle growth are the type 2As—the fibers that are fast-twitch, with an endurance element.

The programs are easy to follow within these pages. The Publishers has taken all guess work out to make this an easy muscle-building experience. Our program stimulate and develop the endurance fast twitch fibers that is important for enhancing muscle growth and increasing power and strength gains.

The programs in this book stress the muscles being worked and not the connective tisses. Development of the hard to reach fibers will not occur unless you keep time under load at 40 plus seconds plus.

Both endurance and anaerobic capabilities are housed with the 2As, so to get the most growth, you need to tax both facets of the muscle for maximum size gains. There will be no low reps by itself within these pages. Low reps build muscle, but growth is slow and limited until the endurance capacities are stimulated. This then stimulates the 2A fast-twitch fibers that promote muscle growth.

This is why the trainee need to stay within the 20 rep range mark, this increases the load time placed on the fibers for serious growth and development to occur. The size principal where low-threshold units are called first to fire, followed by the mediums, then the high threshold units. This is the best way to stimulate many fiber types to fire rapidly within the training plan. This is why the aerobic components are called into play promoting more muscle stimulation and increasing the growth process.

Chapter 2:

CHEST

BUILD A POWERFUL CHEST

BUILD A POWERFUL CHEST

02 BUILD A POWERFUL CHEST

The chest muscles allow you to push or move the arm forward or across the body. These muscles are activated in any throwing or pushing motion. Aesthetically, building a powerful chest is a sign of power in men.

However, the chest muscles are not used daily, so most times they are under developed. So despite, the simplicity of how these muscles contract, they can be trained in a number of various angles of push and pull, each offer its own special muscle enhancing properties.

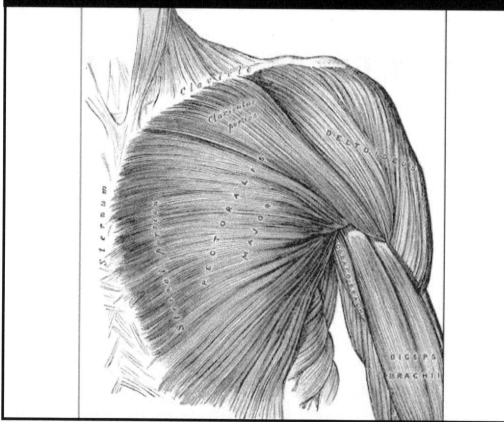

CHEST EXERCISES

02 BUILD A POWERFUL CHEST

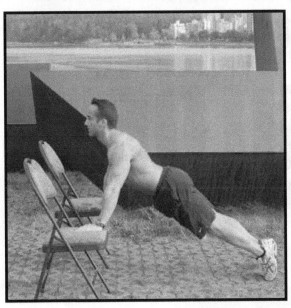

INCLINE PUSHUPS

This exercise is the Granddaddy of all upper-body exercises. It's the best upper-body builder and conditioner there is. This exercise is performed exactly as shown.

Place your hands on two chairs that are 15 inches high, the higher you go the greater pre-stretch there is. At the bottom position to enhance muscle-building stimuli, pause for 2 seconds before reversing the movement.

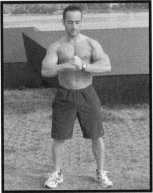

LIEDERMAN PRESS

Start off with the hands at the middle point. Press right palm against the left palm towards the left armpit. Pause 1 second then press the arm back to the other armpit, pause again then repeat.

Chapter 3:

SHOULDERS
DEVELOP POWERFUL SHOULDERS

DEVELOP POWERFUL SHOULDERS

03 DEVELOP POWERFUL SHOULDERS

The shoulder muscles are divided into three heads and are quite unique and move the arm in all directions. The front muscle raise the arm forward, the side muscles made up of a number of muscle bundles, and raises the arm out to the sides. The rear or posterior muscle, is designed to pull the arm backwards. All shoulder exercises are isolation type exercises. They recruit the front and side heads of the shoulders that tie in well with stimulating the upper and mid-back muscles as well giving the entire girdle complete development.

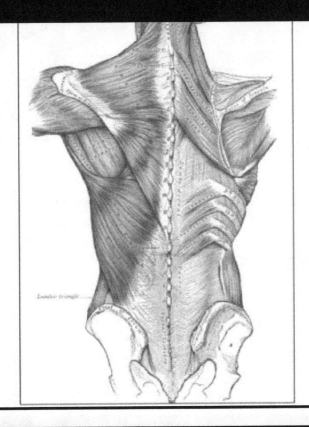

SHOULDER EXERCISES

03 DEVELOP POWERFUL SHOULDERS

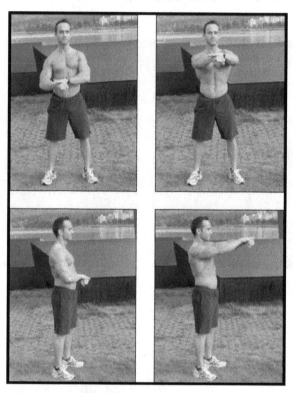

FORWARD RAISES

Grasp the right hand with the left in front of the body as shown. Gradually raise the arm forward against the resistance of the other hand. Repeat for reps then switch arms and continue. This works the Front shoulder muscles.
RESIST IN ONE DIRECTION ONLY

SHOULDER EXERCISES

03 DEVELOP POWERFUL SHOULDERS

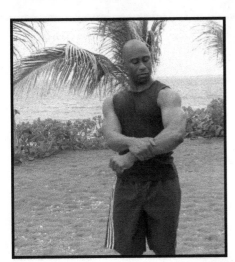 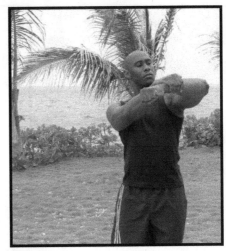

LATERAL RAISES

Grasp the left arm that is across the body as in the picture. Now raise the arm outwards towards the side contracted position resisting with the right arm. Perform desired reps then switch arms. **RESIST IN ONE DIRECTION ONLY**

SHOULDER EXERCISES

03 DEVELOP POWERFUL SHOULDERS

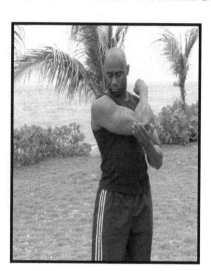 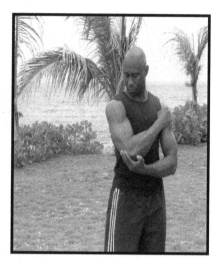

ACROSS THE BODY PULLS

Place Grasp the right elbow as picture shows firmly with the left hand. Slowly force the right elbow downward and backward while resisting with the left hand. Repeat for reps, then switch arms.

This add great strength and development to the (rear) back part of the shoulders, lats and midback. It's best to start with this exercise first for it's easily neglected in a muscle-building program. As they say, out of site out of mind. **RESIST IN ONE DIRECTION ONLY.**

Chapter 4:

UPPER BACK
DEVELOP A POWERFUL V-TAPER

DEVELOP A POWERFUL V-TAPER

04 DEVELOP A POWERFUL V-TAPER

The entire back is made up of many muscles overlapping each other. However most trainees find the back quite difficult to fully develop. The reason? As the saying goes out of sight, out of mind. We cannot directly see the back muscles, plus we cannot see it flex like we would see the biceps.

We make training the entire back musculature much easier making developing the back obviously simple once you know what you are doing, you can bring these muscles up to speed. We are looking at the large Latissimus that covers the majority of the back. The trapezius is broken up into two sections.

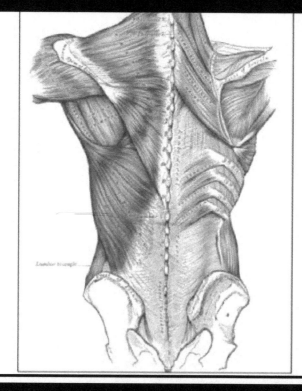

UPPER BACK EXERCISES

04 DEVELOP A POWERFUL V-TAPER

DO NOT NEGLECT THE MID AND LOWER TRAPS

The upper traps and mid-back muscles. Plus, we have the teres major, which is strongly stimulated with unilateral work, which makes self resistance the ideal movement. The infraspinatus muscle is like a half circle on each side of the upper back and is a very important rotator cuff muscle.

This muscle stabilizes the shoulder and prevents dislocations. Even though this muscle is at the back, most traditional exercises do not fully target these muscles. However, with self resistance there are exercises that target this area for full development.

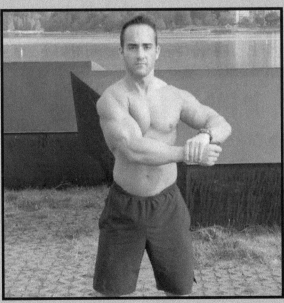

UPPER BACK EXERCISES

04 DEVELOP A POWERFUL V-TAPER

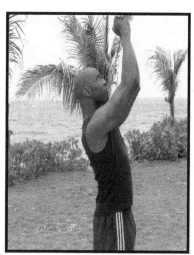 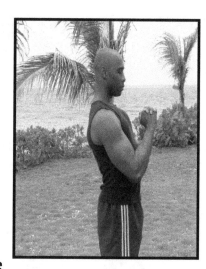

PULLDOWNS

With the arms overhead place your left hand on top of the right fist as shown. Pull down with the left hand resisting with the right, once at finished position press the right hand up resisting with the left hand for the desired reps. Then switch arms. This works the entire upper back and biceps.
RESIST IN ONE DIRECTION ONLY

UPPER BACK EXERCISES

04 DEVELOP A POWERFUL V-TAPER

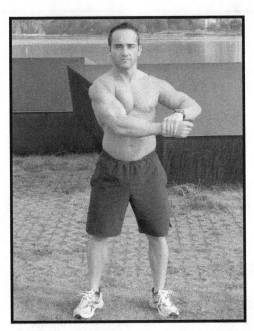 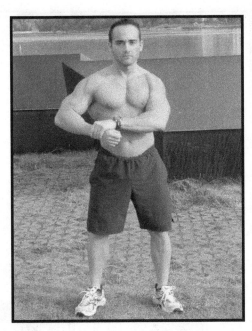

UPPER BACK ROWS

Bring your arm across the body pre-stretching the mid-back, grasp the hand as shown. Slowly pull the arm across the body toward the armpit against the resistance supplied by the other arm. Repeat the movement, then switch arms. This adds thickens to the mid-back, lats, along with the rear part of the shoulders. **RESIST IN ONE DIRECTION ONLY.**

UPPER BACK EXERCISES

04 DEVELOP A POWERFUL V-TAPER

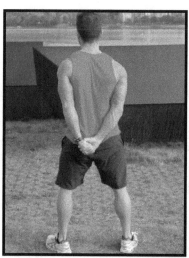 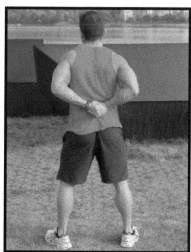

REVERSE UPRIGHT ROWS

ADD POWER TO THE REAR DELT MUSCLES

Place your arm behind your back as shown, hold onto the wrist with the other hand lean forward a-little and pull the right arm upwards while resisting with the right. When fatigue switch arms and continue. This works the mid-back,upper traps and rear delts. **RESIST IN ONE DIRECTION ONLY**

Chapter 5:

BICEPS

DEVELOP POWERFUL BICEPS

DEVELOP POWERFUL BICEPS

05 DEVELOP POWERFUL BICEPS

The biceps muscle has two heads. A short head, which is on the inside of the arm, and a long head, which is on the outside. This is the part that people see first. The main roll of the biceps is to flex the forearm by bringing the hand towards the shoulder. In order to build powerful complete biceps, you need to learn that the biceps do not work by itself.

The brachialis, which is under the bicep when developed, gives the bicep a larger and fuller appearance. Performing curls place undesirable tension on the tendon near the elbow. In other words, the biceps is placed in a very vulnerable position. Always start all bicep exercises with a slight bend at the start and finish. Always maintain tension on the biceps and not the joint.

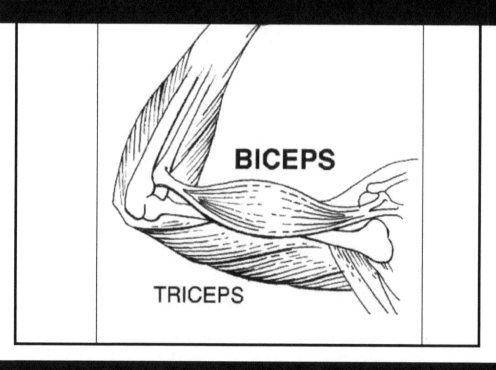

BICEP EXERCISES

05 DEVELOP POWERFUL BICEPS

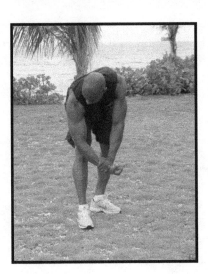 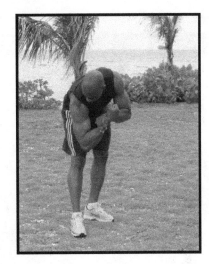

CONCENTRATION CURLS

As pictured, pull the right arm towards the face while resisting with the left hand. Now reverse the exercise by pushing the left arm down and resisting with the right. Complete your reps then switch arms and repeat movement. **DUAL ACTION**

BICEP EXERCISES

05 DEVELOP POWERFUL BICEPS

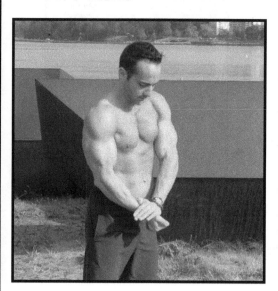 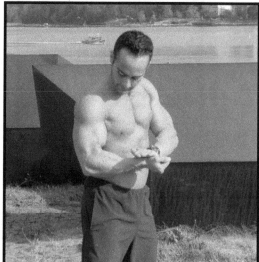

PALM UP CURLS

Pull the right arm upward towards the shoulder while resisting with the left hand. At the shoulder, reverse the exercise by pushing the left arm downwards, resisting with the right. **DUAL ACTION**

Chapter 6:

TRICEPS
DEVELOP POWERFUL TRICEPS

DEVELOP POWERFUL TRICEPS

06 DEVELOP POWERFUL TRICEPS

DEVELOP POWERFUL TRICEPS

The triceps has three heads: The lateral head, middle head and the long head. The role of the triceps is to straighten the arm. The triceps work in opposition to the biceps and brachialis muscles. The triceps has three heads this makes it much larger in mass than the biceps and the brachialis.

Unfortunately, most pay attention to the biceps, leaving the triceps underdeveloped. The lateral head, which is on the outside is what people see first. The triceps are easy to develop and we have made it easy for the trainee to achieve this.

TRICEP EXERCISES

06 DEVELOP POWERFUL TRICEPS

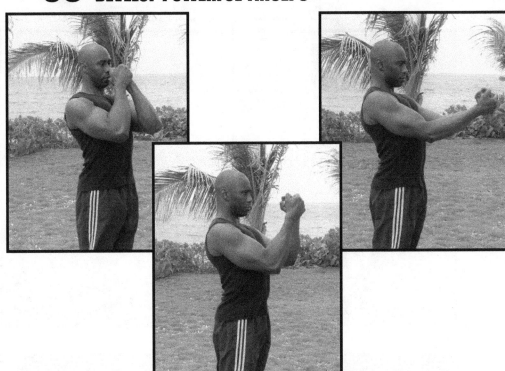

FORWARD EXTENSIONS

As shown above, press the left arm forward while resisting with the right hand. **Do not straighten the elbow.**
RESIST IN A DUAL MANNER

TRICEP EXERCISES

06 DEVELOP POWERFUL TRICEPS

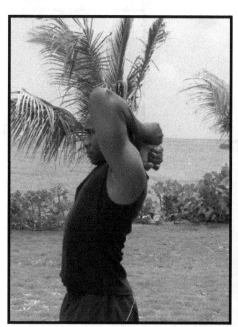 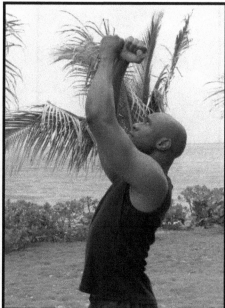

OVERHEAD TRICEP EXTENSIONS

Place arms overhead, press the right arm upwards while resisting with the left arm. Use a light to moderate tension due to the tricep tendons being sensitive at that position. **Do not straighten the elbow. RESIST IN ONE DIRECTION ONLY**

TRICEP EXERCISES

06 DEVELOP POWERFUL TRICEPS

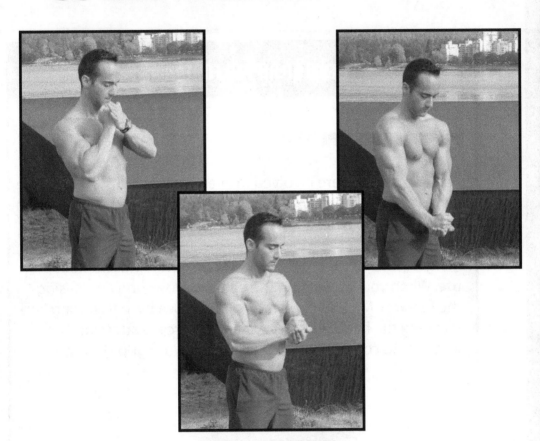

TRICEP PRESSDOWN

As pictured above, press the right hand downwards while resisting with the left arm. Repeat desired reps then switch arms. **RESIST IN ONE DIRECTION ONLY**

DEVELOP RIPPED FOREARMS

07 DEVELOP RIPPED FOREARMS

DEVELOP RIPPED FOREARMS

DEVELOP RIPPED FOREARMS

Forearm muscles are involved in every daily activity, just like the calves and abdominals. We use these muscles all the time, when we drive, write, type, hold a bag and even open a door.

Many of the muscles of the forearm deal with Muscle-multi-use. When you are moving the elbow by lowering and raising the forearm. Moving the wrist up and down by, plus raising and lowering the hand. All self resistance exercises stress the forearms to contract which will increase your grip strength.

FOREARM EXERCISES

07 DEVELOP RIPPED FOREARMS

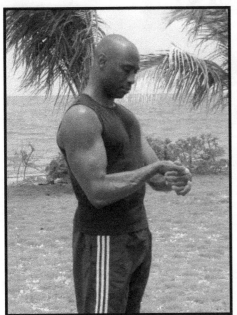

EXERCISE ONE

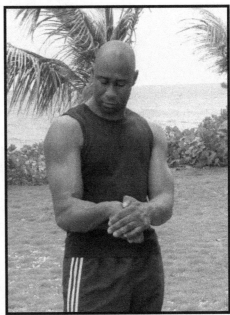

EXERCISE TWO

HAND/FOREARM EXERCISE

EXERCISE ONE: As pictured press the right hand upwards until the fingers are pointed towards you. Return to position and repeat. **RESIST IN ONE DIRECTION**

EXERCISE TWO: Same as exercise one but, the hand is placed downwards.

Chapter 8:

THIGHS
DEVELOP POWERFUL THIGHS

DEVELOP POWERFUL TIRELESS THIGHS

08 DEVELOP POWERFUL TIRELESS THIGHS

DEVELOP POWERFUL THIGHS

The thigh muscles are basically made up of four main muscles: the vastus lateral muscle, this is located on the outside of the thighs. The vastus medial muscle, this is located on the inside of the thigh muscles towards the knee.

Better known as the tear drop because of its shape. The recus-femoris, which is located in the center of the muscles, and the vastus intermedius, this muscle is mostly covered by all the other muscles of the thighs. This program Develop tireless thighs with a power pack punch.

LEG EXERCISES

08 DEVELOP POWERFUL TIRELESS THIGHS

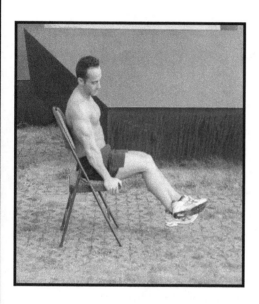 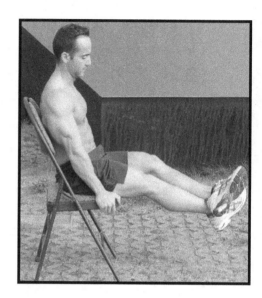

LEG EXTENSIONS

While seated on a chair, box or stool, place the legs as shown in the picture. Now extend the left leg outwards resisting with the right. At the top pause for 2 seconds, then reverse the movement by pulling down with the right while resisting with the left. **DO NOT STRAIGHTEN THE KNEE. RESIST IN A DUAL MANNER**

LEG EXERCISES

08 DEVELOP POWERFUL TIRELESS THIGHS

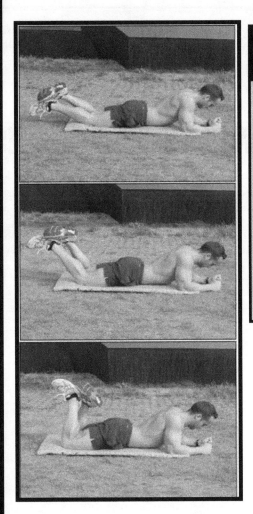

LEG CURL

As shown, pull the right leg towards the lower back, powerfully resisting with the left leg. At the finished position, press the left foot down resisting with the right.

PERFORM IN A DUAL MANNER

Chapter 9:

LOWER BACK
DEVELOP POWERFUL LOWER-BACK MUSCLES

DEVELOP POWERFUL LOWER BACK MUSCLES

09 DEVELOP POWERFUL LOWER-BACK MUSCLES

POWERFUL LOWER BACK MUSCLES

Develop Powerful Lower back muscles
The lower back muscles support the lower part of the spine. When these muscles are well developed it builds a brace protecting the spine.

Apart from that the lower back muscles are responsible for bringing the body upright from a leaning forward position. Not only will the lower back be involved, but the glutes and hamstrings come into play.

LOWER BACK EXERCISES

09 DEVELOP POWERFUL LOWER BACK

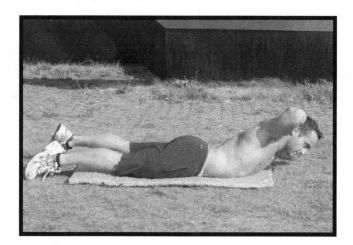

LOWER BACK EXTENSION

As shown above, this is the finished position. Lay flat on the floor and perform this movement by raising the upper body upwards slowly pause for 2 seconds at the top. Then slowly reverse the movement under control.

Chapter 10:

CALVES
DEVELOP SHAPELY CALVES

DEVELOP SHAPELY CALVES

10 DEVELOP SHAPELY CALVES

DEVELOP SHAPELY CALVES

Develop shapely calves

The calves add a finished look to the lower leg with a diamond shape. This muscle has three heads (muscle parts) the soleus, this is under the large lateral head and gives the calves a fully developed look viewed from the side and back.

The lateral and medial heads are on the outside and in the middle of the muscle. The gastrocnemius make up the majority of the calf muscle. However, the longer the gastroc, the larger the potential for enhanced calf muscle development. With the stretch component this adds strength, shape and muscle development in double quick time.

DEVELOP SHAPELY CALVES

10 DEVELOP SHAPELY CALVES

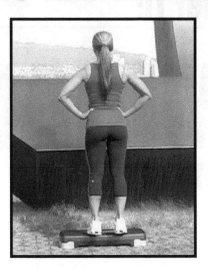 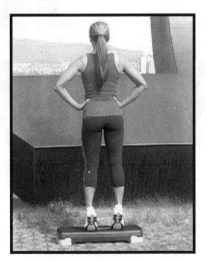

STANDING CALVE RAISES

Position yourself as shown but make sure the calves are well stretched. Start off as shown in the picture start position. Press straight up on the toes then lower. This is as awesome calve stretch exercise. Perform this exercise until the calves are well tired. This stimulates the entire calve.

Chapter 11:

ABDOMINALS
DEVELOP RIPPED ABS

DEVELOP RIPPED ABS

11 DEVELOP RIPPED ABS

The abdominal muscles are very important and reveal that the trainee has a lean physique. Plus, the role of the abdominal muscles is to protect the spine. A lean chiseled set of abdominal muscles shows the opposite sex that the owner has a sign of virility.

Once these muscles are well developed this keeps the waist line and belly flat. There are various muscle structures that complete the overall look, the entire length of the abdominal wall, plus the internal and external obliques.

The lower sections of the abdominal muscles play the largest role in protecting the spine and storing belly fat. This is the easiest place for body-fat to accumulate. Which makes training with self resistance the ideal exercise to attack those muscle fibers to the maximum.

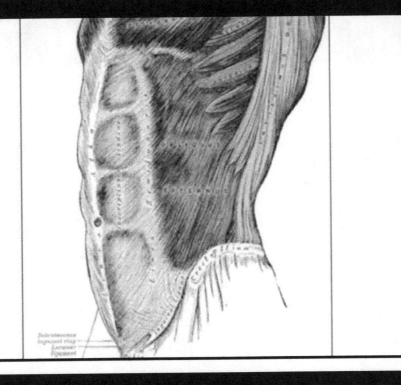

DEVELOP RIPPED ABS

11 DEVELOP RIPPED ABS

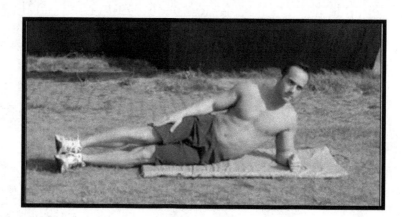

DEVELOP RIPPED ABDOMINALS

As noted in the introduction the abdominal wall includes four muscles: Let's cover the entire length from the chest to pubis is called the rectus abdominis, people say abs for short. The abdominal wall should be worked in three angles of flexion. The lower sections of the abdominal muscles. The upper sections of the abdominal wall, and the obliques. Which are rotator muscles.

DEVELOP RIPPED ABS

11 DEVELOP RIPPED ABS

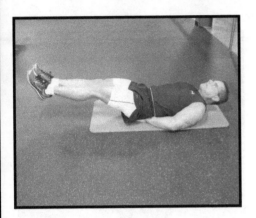 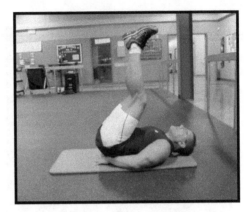

REVERSE CRUNCHES

As shown above, place your hands under your butt slowly raise the legs upwards towards the chest or stomach. Pause for a1 second count then slowly reverse the movement. This exercise stimulates the entire abdominal wall.

DEVELOP RIPPED ABS

11 DEVELOP RIPPED ABS

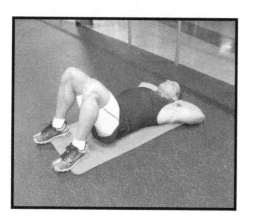 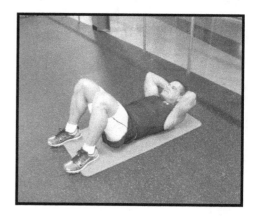

ABDOMINAL CRUNCHES

Lay on your back. Place the hands at your ear, tilt your head back, focus on the ceiling and crunch upward as shown.
DO NOT PULL ON THE HEAD.

Chapter 12:

THE ULTIMATE FIBER SURGE METHOD

REP SPEED 2 SECONDS CONTRACTED 2 SECONDS RELEASE.
ALL BODY-WEIGHT MOVES PERFORM 20 REPS EACH
ALL PHASES ARE TO BE PERFORMED FOR 4 WEEKS DO NOT SKIP PHASES

FIBER SURGE PHASE ONE

12 FIBER SURGE METHOD

MONDAY, WEDNESDAY, FRIDAY

Perform 15 reps each movement before moving to the next exercise. On the 15th rep perform a 10 second Isometric contraction at the middle of the exercise stroke. When the full cycle is completed, perform another round if needed. Perform each exercise using 50% of force.

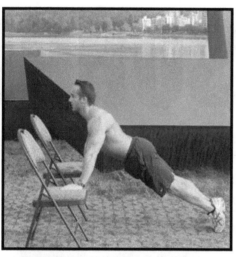
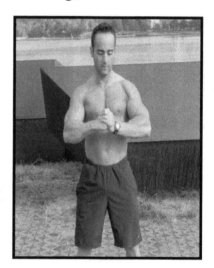
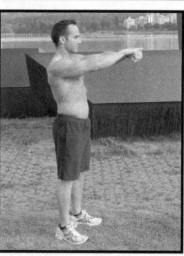
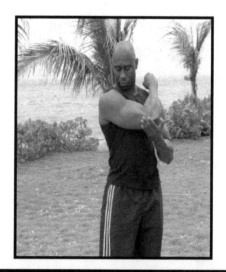

FIBER SURGE PHASE ONE

12 FIBER SURGE METHOD

MONDAY, WEDNESDAY, FRIDAY
Routine continued.........

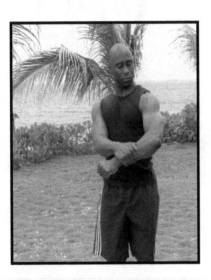

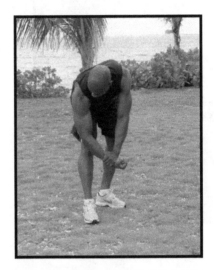

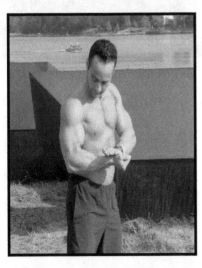

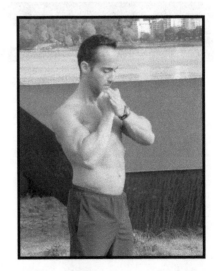

FIBER SURGE PHASE ONE

12 FIBER SURGE METHOD

MONDAY, WEDNESDAY, FRIDAY
Routine continued...........

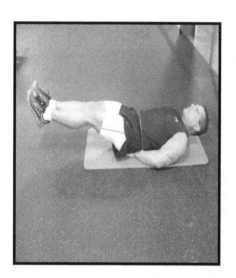 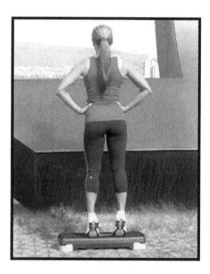

PHASE ONE MON, WED, FRI

FIBER SURGE PHASE ONE

12 FIBER SURGE METHOD

TUESDAY, THURSDAY, SATURDAY

Perform 15 reps before moving to the next exercise. On the 15th rep perform a 10 second Isometric contraction at the middle of the exercise stroke. When the full cycle is completed, perform another round if needed. Perform each exercise using 50% of force.

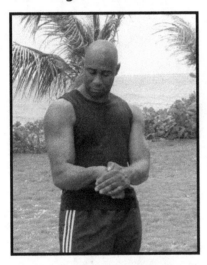
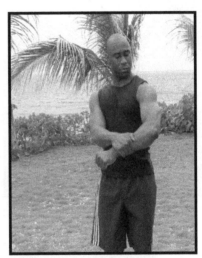
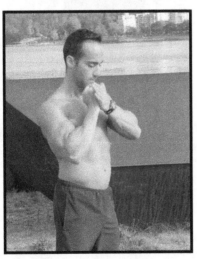
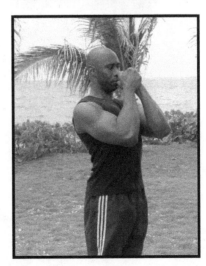

FIBER SURGE PHASE ONE

12 FIBER SURGE METHOD

TUESDAY, THURSDAY, SATURDAY
Continued routine..........

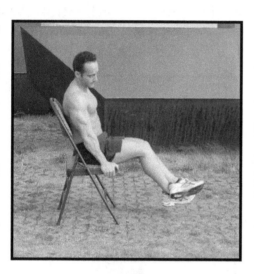

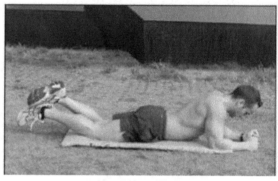

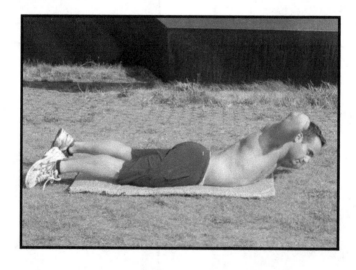

FIBER SURGE PHASE ONE

12 FIBER SURGE METHOD

TUESDAY, THURSDAY, SATURDAY
Continued routine........

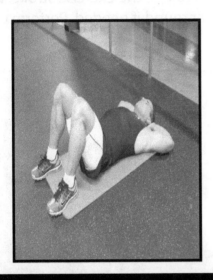 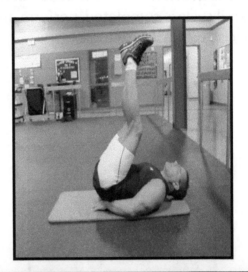

PHASE ONE TUES, THURS, SAT.

PHASE TWO

13 FIBER SURGE METHOD

MONDAY, WEDNESDAY, FRIDAY
Perform 5-7 reps before moving to the next exercise. On the 7th rep perform a 10 second Isometric contraction at the middle of the exercise stroke. When the full cycle is completed, perform another round if needed. Perform each exercise using 50% of force.

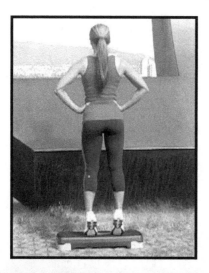
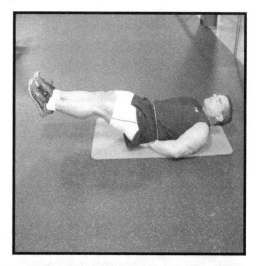
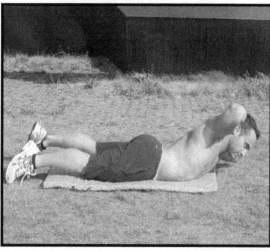
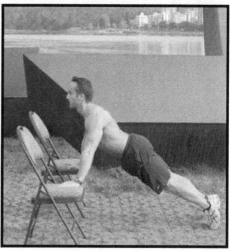

PHASE TWO

13 FIBER SURGE METHOD

**MONDAY, WEDNESDAY, FRIDAY
ROUTINE CONTINUED........**

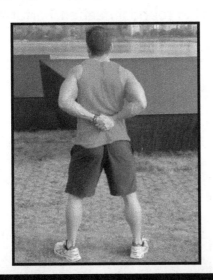
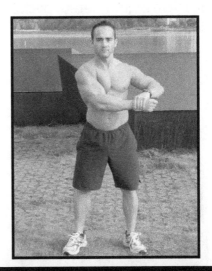

PHASE TWO   MON, WED, FRI.

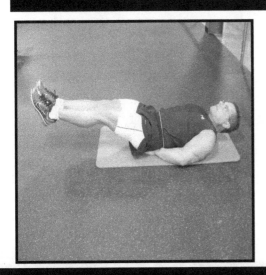
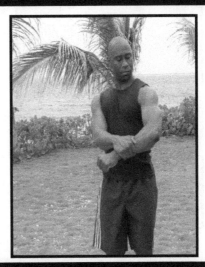

PHASE TWO

13 FIBER SURGE METHOD

TUESDAY, THURSDAY, SATURDAY

Perform 5-7 reps before moving to the next exercise. On the 7th rep perform a 10 second Isometric contraction at the middle of the exercise stroke. When the full cycle is completed, perform another round if needed. Perform each exercise using 50% of force.

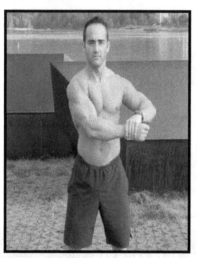 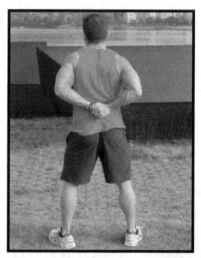

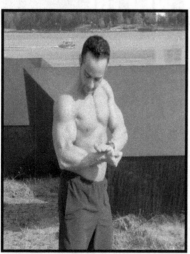 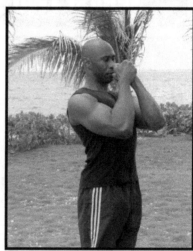

PHASE TWO

13 FIBER SURGE METHOD

TUESDAY, THURSDAY, SATURDAY

ROUTINE CONTINUED..........

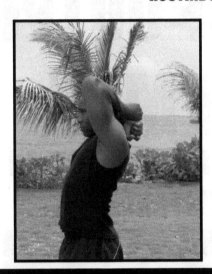 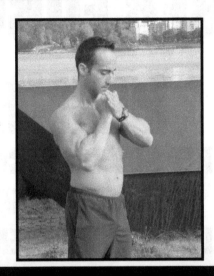

PHASE TWO   TUES, THURS, SAT.

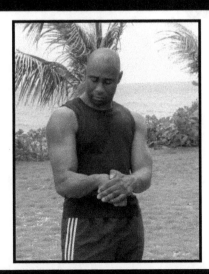 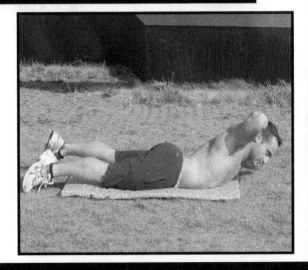

Chapter 14:

FIBER FORCE OUTPUT POWER MAX

REP SPEED 2 SECOND CONTRACTION
6 SECOND RELEASE
ALL BODYWEIGHT EXERCISES PERFORM
20 REPS EACH
4 WEEKS

POWER MAX

14 POWER MAX METHOD

HOW TO PERFORM THIS ROUTINE:

Perform 5 reps before moving to the next exercise. On the 5th rep perform a 7 second Isometric contraction at the middle of the exercise stroke. Perform one set each exercise using 50% of force.

DAY ONE

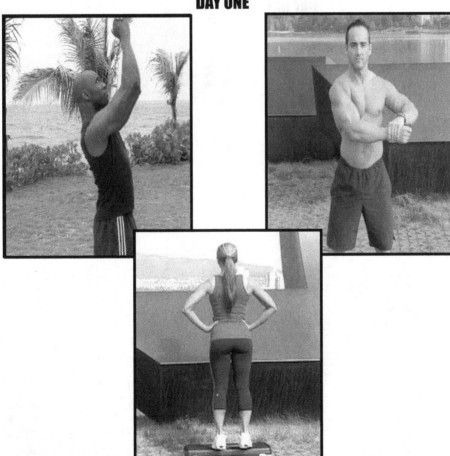

POWER MAX

14 POWER MAX METHOD

HOW TO PERFORM THIS ROUTINE:

Perform 5 reps before moving to the next exercise. On the 5th rep perform a 7 second Isometric contraction at the middle of the exercise stroke. Perform one set each exercise using 50% of force.

DAY ONE continued..........

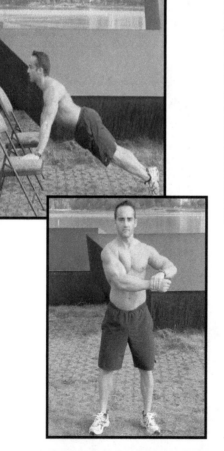

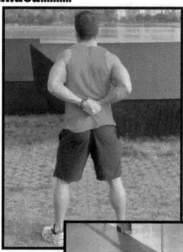

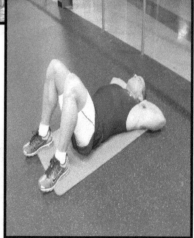

POWER MAX

14 POWER MAX METHOD

HOW TO PERFORM THIS ROUTINE:
Perform 5 reps before moving to the next exercise. On the 5th rep perform a 7 second Isometric contraction at the middle of the exercise stroke. Perform one set each exercise using 50% of force.

DAY TWO

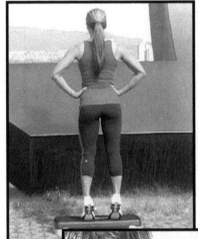

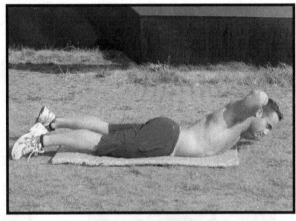

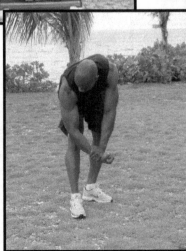

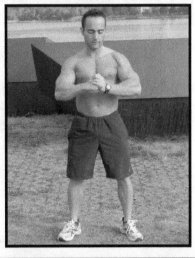

POWER MAX

14 POWER MAX METHOD

HOW TO PERFORM THIS ROUTINE:

Perform 5 reps before moving to the next exercise. On the 5th rep perform a 7 second Isometric contraction at the middle of the exercise stroke. Perform one set each exercise using 50% of force.

DAY TWO continued............

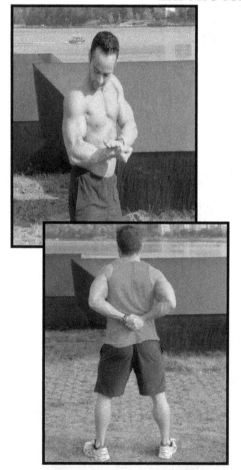

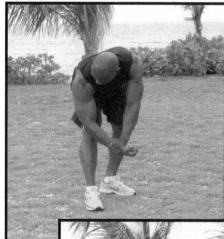

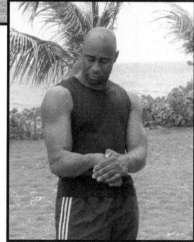

POWER MAX

14 POWER MAX METHOD

HOW TO PERFORM THIS ROUTINE:

Perform 5 reps before moving to the next exercise. On the 5th rep perform a 7 second Isometric contraction at the middle of the exercise stroke. Perform one set each exercise using 50% of force.

DAY THREE

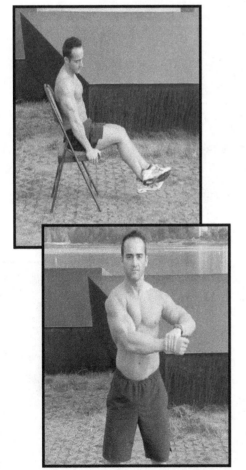

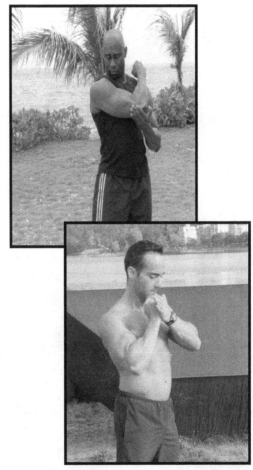

POWER MAX

14 POWER MAX METHOD

HOW TO PERFORM THIS ROUTINE:

Perform 5 reps before moving to the next exercise. On the 5th rep perform a 7 second Isometric contraction at the middle of the exercise stroke. Perform one set each exercise using 50% of force.

DAY THREE continued.......

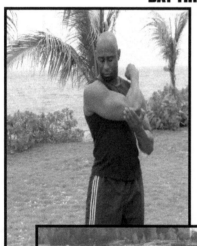

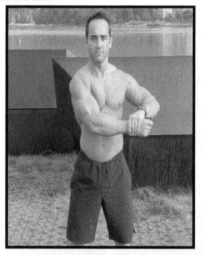

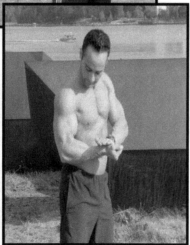

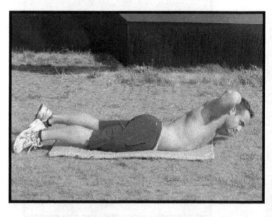

POWER MAX

14 POWER MAX METHOD

HOW TO PERFORM THIS ROUTINE:

Perform 5 reps before moving to the next exercise. On the 5th rep perform a 7 second Isometric contraction at the middle of the exercise stroke. Perform one set each exercise using 50% of force.

DAY THREE continued.......

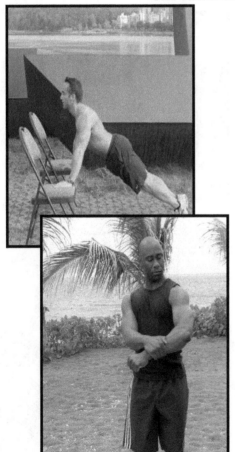

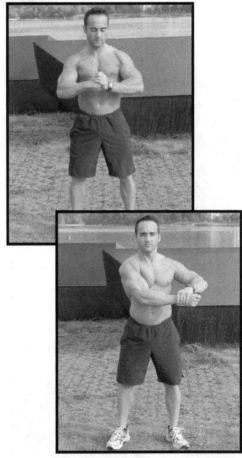

POWER MAX

14 POWER MAX METHOD

HOW TO PERFORM THIS ROUTINE:
Perform 5 reps before moving to the next exercise. On the 5th rep perform a 7 second Isometric contraction at the middle of the exercise stroke. Perform one set each exercise using 50% of force.

DAY FOUR

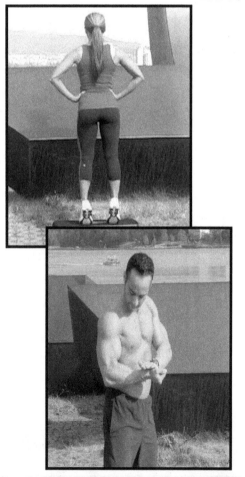
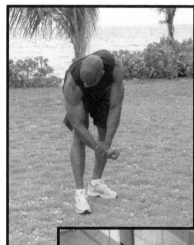
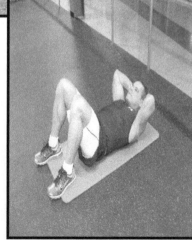

POWER MAX

14 POWER MAX METHOD

HOW TO PERFORM THIS ROUTINE:
Perform 5 reps before moving to the next exercise. On the 5th rep perform a 7 second Isometric contraction at the middle of the exercise stroke. Perform one set each exercise using 50% of force.

DAY FOUR continued......

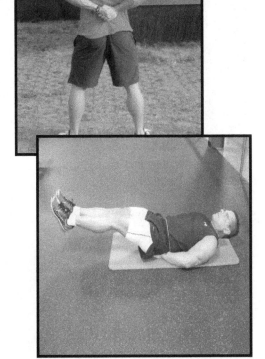
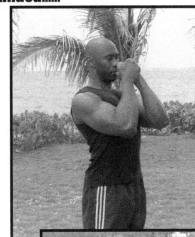
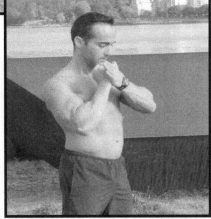

POWER MAX

14 POWER MAX METHOD

HOW TO PERFORM THIS ROUTINE:
Perform 5 reps before moving to the next exercise. On the 5th rep perform a 7 second Isometric contraction at the middle of the exercise stroke. Perform one set each exercise using 50% of force.

DAY FIVE

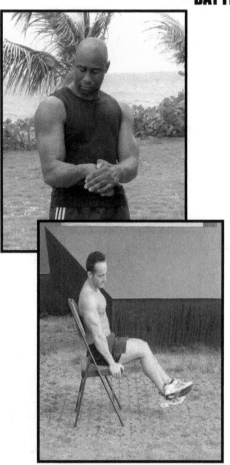

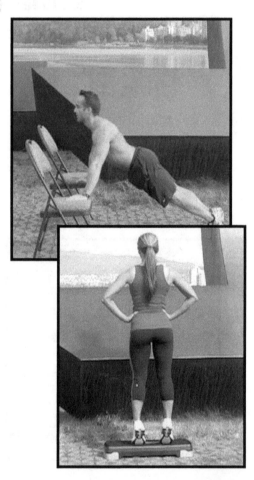

POWER MAX

14 POWER MAX METHOD

HOW TO PERFORM THIS ROUTINE:

Perform 5 reps before moving to the next exercise. On the 5th rep perform a 7 second Isometric contraction at the middle of the exercise stroke. Perform one set each exercise using 50% of force.

DAY FIVE continued.....

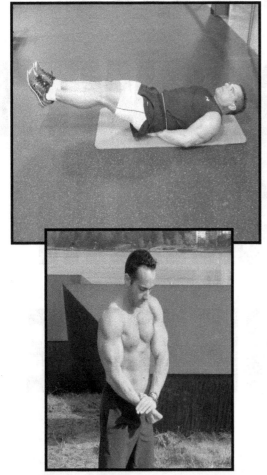

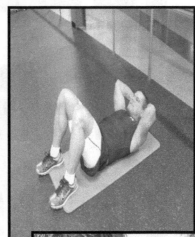

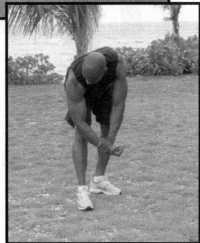

Chapter 15:

THE ISOTONIC MAX-GROWTH PROGRAM PHASE ONE

THE ISOTONIC MAX-GROWTH PROGRAM

15 THE ISOTONIC MAX-GROWTH PROGRAM

HOW TO PERFORM THIS ROUTINE:
PHASE ONE
Perform 7 full reps, followed by 15 reps from the start to middle point of the exercise stroke. On the 15th rep perform a 30 second isometric contraction. One set per exercise. **REP SPEED 2 SECONDS CONTRACTED, 2 SECONDS RELEASE**

DAY ONE

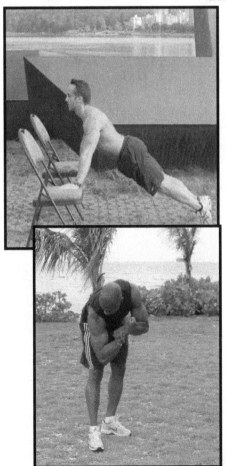
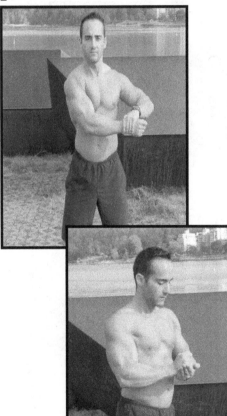

THE ISOTONIC MAX-GROWTH PROGRAM

15 THE ISOTONIC MAX-GROWTH PROGRAM

HOW TO PERFORM THIS ROUTINE:
PHASE ONE

Perform 7 full reps, followed by 15 reps from the start to middle point of the exercise stroke. On the 15th rep perform a 30 second isometric contraction. One set per exercise. **REP SPEED 2 SECONDS CONTRACTED, 2 SECONDS RELEASE**

DAY ONE continued............

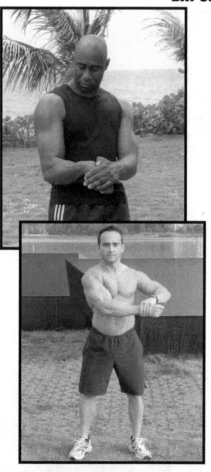

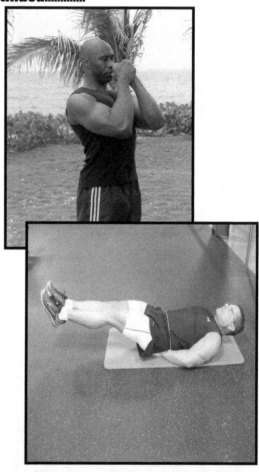

THE ISOTONIC MAX-GROWTH PROGRAM

15   THE ISOTONIC MAX-GROWTH PROGRAM

HOW TO PERFORM THIS ROUTINE:
PHASE ONE

Perform 7 full reps, followed by 15 reps from the start to middle point of the exercise stroke. On the 15th rep perform a 30 second isometric contraction. One set per exercise. **REP SPEED 2 SECONDS CONTRACTED, 2 SECONDS RELEASE**

DAY TWO

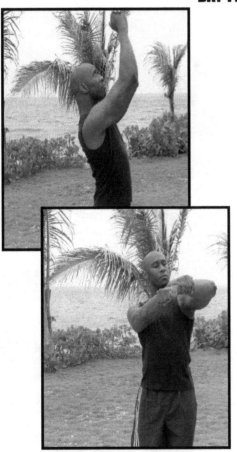

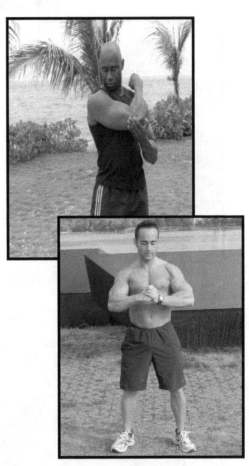

THE ISOTONIC MAX-GROWTH PROGRAM

15 THE ISOTONIC MAX-GROWTH PROGRAM

HOW TO PERFORM THIS ROUTINE:
PHASE ONE

Perform 7 full reps, followed by 15 reps from the start to middle point of the exercise stroke. On the 15th rep perform a 30 second isometric contraction. One set per exercise. **REP SPEED 2 SECONDS CONTRACTED, 2 SECONDS RELEASE**

DAY TWO continued.......

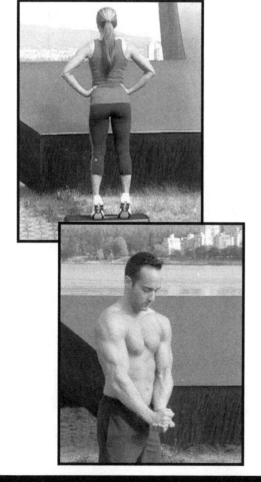

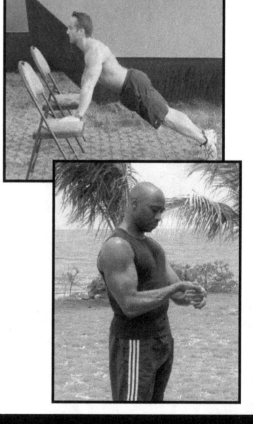

THE ISOTONIC MAX-GROWTH PROGRAM

15 THE ISOTONIC MAX-GROWTH PROGRAM

HOW TO PERFORM THIS ROUTINE:
PHASE ONE

Perform 7 full reps, followed by 15 reps from the start to middle point of the exercise stroke. On the 15th rep perform a 30 second isometric contraction. One set per exercise. **REP SPEED 2 SECONDS CONTRACTED, 2 SECONDS RELEASE**

DAY THREE

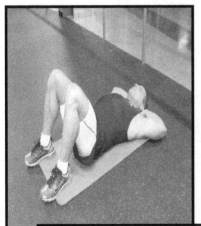

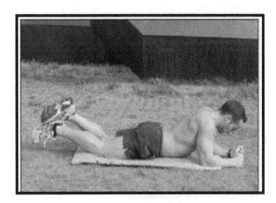

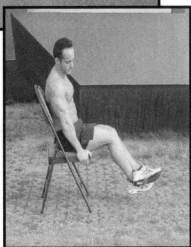

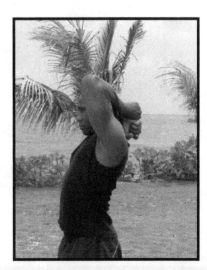

THE ISOTONIC MAX-GROWTH PROGRAM

15 THE ISOTONIC MAX-GROWTH PROGRAM

HOW TO PERFORM THIS ROUTINE:
PHASE ONE

Perform 7 full reps, followed by 15 reps from the start to middle point of the exercise stroke. On the 15th rep perform a 30 second isometric contraction. One set per exercise. **REP SPEED 2 SECONDS CONTRACTED, 2 SECONDS RELEASE**

DAY THREE continued..........

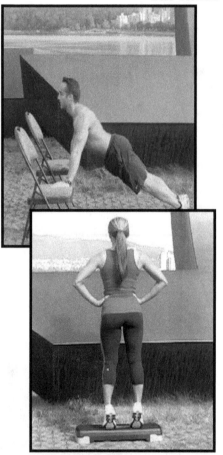

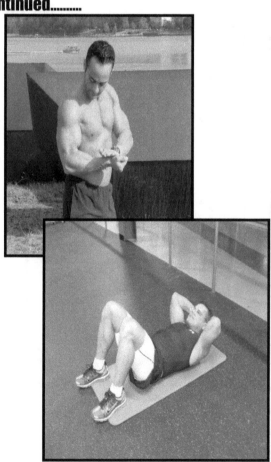

THE ISOTONIC MAX-GROWTH PROGRAM

15 THE ISOTONIC MAX-GROWTH PROGRAM

HOW TO PERFORM THIS ROUTINE:
PHASE ONE

Perform 7 full reps, followed by 15 reps from the start to middle point of the exercise stroke. On the 15th rep perform a 30 second isometric contraction. One set per exercise. **REP SPEED 2 SECONDS CONTRACTED, 2 SECONDS RELEASE**

DAY FOUR

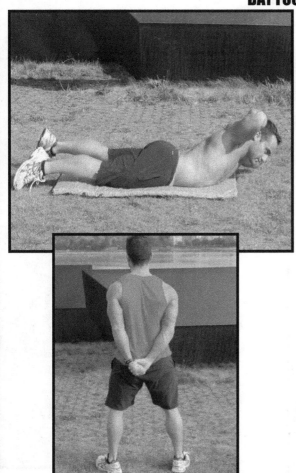

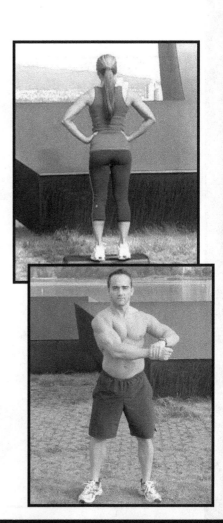

THE ISOTONIC MAX-GROWTH PROGRAM

15 THE ISOTONIC MAX-GROWTH PROGRAM

HOW TO PERFORM THIS ROUTINE:
PHASE ONE
Perform 7 full reps, followed by 15 reps from the start to middle point of the exercise stroke. On the 15th rep perform a 30 second isometric contraction. One set per exercise. **REP SPEED 2 SECONDS CONTRACTED, 2 SECONDS RELEASE**

DAY FIVE

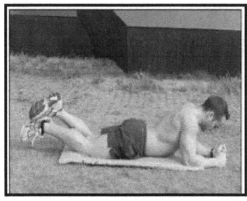

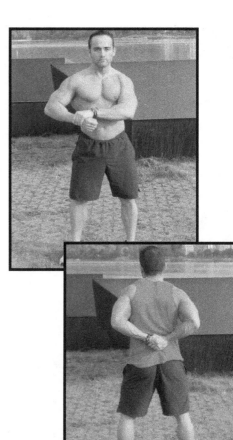

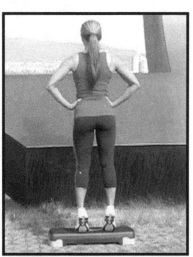

THE ISOTONIC MAX-GROWTH PROGRAM

15 THE ISOTONIC MAX-GROWTH PROGRAM

HOW TO PERFORM THIS ROUTINE:
PHASE ONE
Perform 7 full reps, followed by 15 reps from the start to middle point of the exercise stroke. On the 15th rep perform a 30 second isometric contraction. One set per exercise. **REP SPEED 2 SECONDS CONTRACTED, 2 SECONDS RELEASE**

DAY FIVE continued............

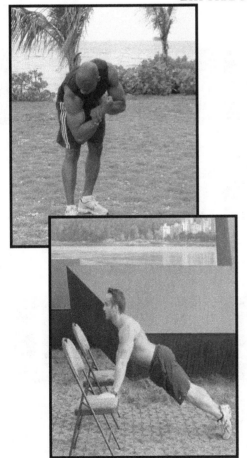

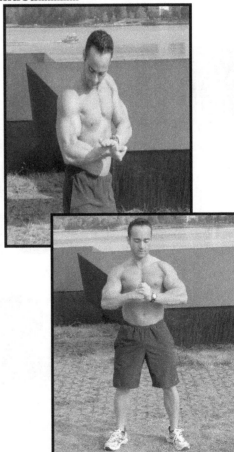

Chapter 15:

THE ISOTONIC MAX-GROWTH PROGRAM PHASE TWO

THE ISOTONIC MAX-GROWTH PROGRAM

15 THE ISOTONIC MAX-GROWTH PROGRAM

HOW TO PERFORM THIS ROUTINE:
PHASE TWO

Contract within 2 seconds then slowly reverse the movement for 6 seconds. Perform 3 reps. On the 3th rep perform an isometric hold for 10 seconds. Alternate day one and day two for 6 days per week. One set per exercise. **Perform this program for 4 weeks**.

DAY ONE

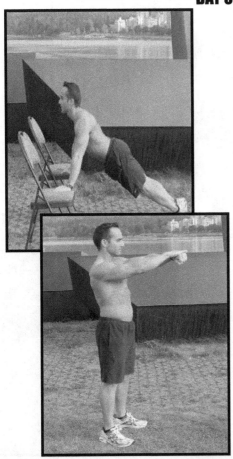

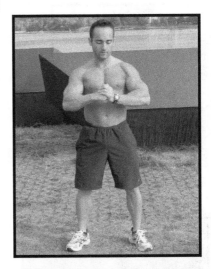

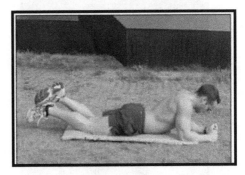

THE ISOTONIC MAX-GROWTH PROGRAM

15 THE ISOTONIC MAX-GROWTH PROGRAM

HOW TO PERFORM THIS ROUTINE:
PHASE TWO

Contract within 2 seconds then slowly reverse the movement for 6 seconds. Perform 3 reps. On the 3th rep perform an isometric hold for 10 seconds. Alternate day one and day two for 6 days per week. One set per exercise. **Perform this program for 4 weeks**.

DAY ONE continued.........

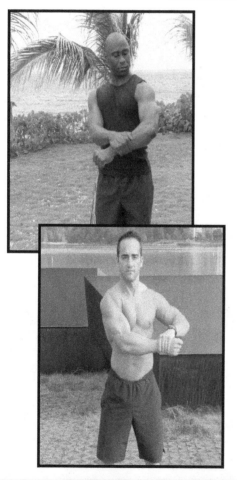

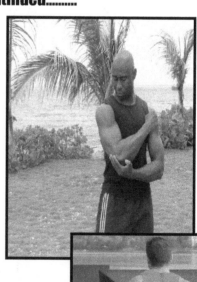

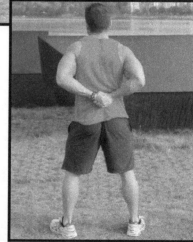

THE ISOTONIC MAX-GROWTH PROGRAM

15 THE ISOTONIC MAX-GROWTH PROGRAM

HOW TO PERFORM THIS ROUTINE:
PHASE TWO

Contract within 2 seconds then slowly reverse the movement for 6 seconds. Perform 3 reps. On the 3th rep perform an isometric hold for 10 seconds. Alternate day one and day two for 6 days per week. One set per exercise. **Perform this program for 4 weeks**.

DAY TWO

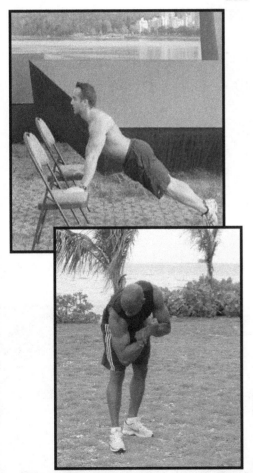

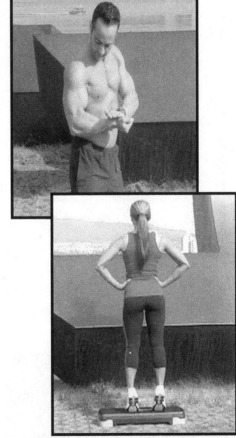

THE ISOTONIC MAX-GROWTH PROGRAM

15 THE ISOTONIC MAX-GROWTH PROGRAM

HOW TO PERFORM THIS ROUTINE:
PHASE TWO
Contract within 2 seconds then slowly reverse the movement for 6 seconds. Perform 3 reps. On the 3th rep perform an isometric hold for 10 seconds. Alternate day one and day two for 6 days per week. One set per exercise. **Perform this program for 4 weeks**.

DAY TWO continued........

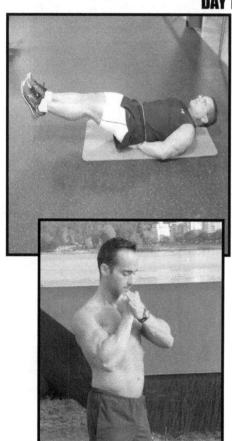

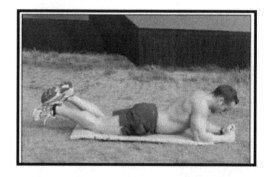

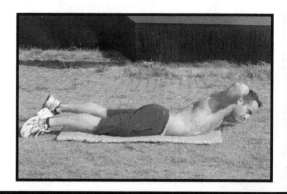

Chapter 15:

THE ISOTONIC MAX-GROWTH PROGRAM PHASE THREE

THE ISOTONIC MAX-GROWTH PROGRAM

15 THE ISOTONIC MAX-GROWTH PROGRAM

HOW TO PERFORM THIS ROUTINE:
PHASE THREE

Perform 20 full reps —by contracting for 2 seconds and release 2 seconds. On the 20th rep perform 10 half reps, start to mid-point. Alternate day one and day two for 6 days per week. **1-2 ROUNDS**

DAY ONE

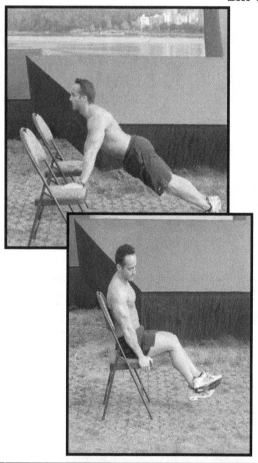

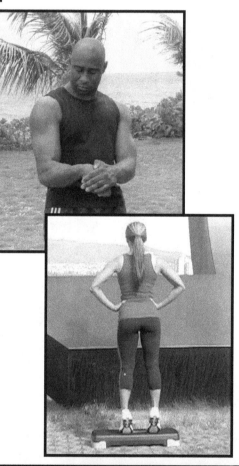

THE ISOTONIC MAX-GROWTH PROGRAM

15 THE ISOTONIC MAX-GROWTH PROGRAM

HOW TO PERFORM THIS ROUTINE:
PHASE THREE
Perform 20 full reps —by contracting for 2 seconds and release 2 seconds. On the 20th rep perform 10 half reps, start to mid-point. Alternate day one and day two for 6 days per week. **1-2 ROUNDS**

DAY ONE continued...........

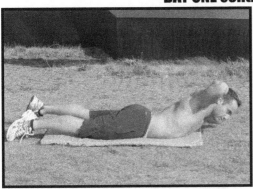

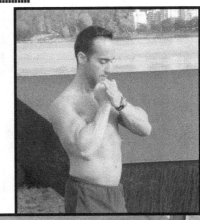

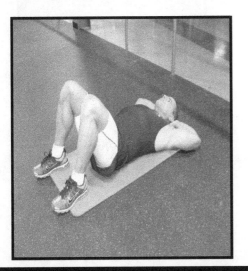

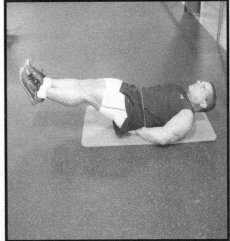

THE ISOTONIC MAX-GROWTH PROGRAM

15 THE ISOTONIC MAX-GROWTH PROGRAM

HOW TO PERFORM THIS ROUTINE:
PHASE THREE

Perform 20 full reps —by contracting for 2 seconds and release 2 seconds. On the 20th rep perform 10 half reps, start to mid-point. Alternate day one and day two for 6 days per week. **1-2 ROUNDS**

DAY TWO

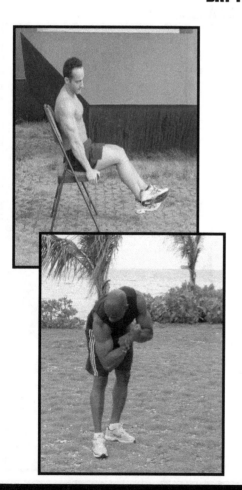

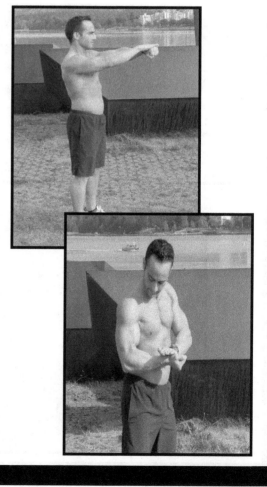

THE ISOTONIC MAX-GROWTH PROGRAM

15 THE ISOTONIC MAX-GROWTH PROGRAM

HOW TO PERFORM THIS ROUTINE:
PHASE THREE

Perform 20 full reps —by contracting for 2 seconds and release 2 seconds. On the 20th rep perform 10 half reps, start to mid-point. Alternate day one and day two for 6 days per week. **1-2 ROUNDS**

DAY TWO continued..........

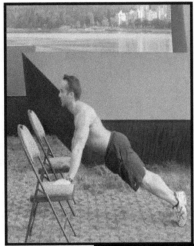
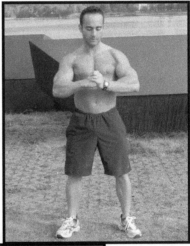

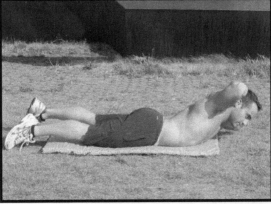

We are looking forward to hearing from you on your progress.
Please drop us an email at.....
greg4vrt@sbcglobal.net or gregm@noram-clutch.com

CPSIA information can be obtained
at www.ICGtesting.com
Printed in the USA
JSHW021410090420
5023JS00005B/819

9 781927 558997